COMING
of
AGE

COMING
of
AGE

The Easy Guide To Healthy
Hair Care for Teens

Keianna Johnson

London Lane Designs and Publishing Services

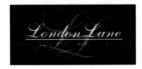

LondonLaneDesigns.com

Copyright © 2018 by Keianna Johnson

All rights reserved. The author and publisher of this book and the accompanying materials have used their best efforts in preparing this book. The author and publisher make no representation or warranties with respect to the accuracy, applicability, fitness, or completeness of the contents of this book. The information contained in this book is strictly for educational purposes. Therefore, if you wish to apply ideas contained in this book, you are taking full responsibility for your actions.

The author and publisher disclaim any warranties (express or implied), merchantability, or fitness for any particular purpose.

The author and publisher shall in no event be held liable to any party for any direct, indirect, punitive, special, incidental or other consequential damages arising directly or indirectly from any use of this material, which is provided "as is", and without warranties. As always, the advice of a competent legal, tax, accounting or other professional should be sought.

This book edition is protected under the US Copyright Act of 1976 and all other applicable international, federal, state and local laws, with ALL rights reserved. No part of this may be copied except for personal use, or changed in any format, sold, or used in any way other than what is outlined within this book except for personal use without express permission from keiannajohnson.com.

DEDICATION

I dedicate this book to my five children. No matter what degrading messages this world may try to make you believe about our Black Lives, History or Culture, know that you are brilliant, and beautiful just the way you are. Your validation isn't in what people say you are; your validation is in who God says you are.

CONT

Table Of Contents

Foreword by Ansylla Ramsey — 1
Introduction — 3
Chapter 1: Natural Hair Care for Teens — 5
Chapter 2: Loc Care for Teens — 19
Chapter 3: Hair Damage: Every Teen's Nightmare — 25
Chapter 4: Trendy Braids & Their Care — 29
Chapter 5: Protecting Your Edges — 37
Chapter 6: Styling Tools & Accessories — 43
Chapter 7: Should Friends Style Your Hair? — 47
Chapter 8: When To Seek A Professional — 49
Chapter 9: Be Encouraged — 53
Chapter 10: Your Hair Diary — 55
Acknowledgments — 69
Resources — 71
About The Author — 73

FOREWARD

I honestly can't recall exactly when I first connected with Keianna Johnson of Chi Chi Sophistication Kids Natural Hair Studio. But when she comes to mind, I always think of her kind spirit and warm smile. When I sought a stylist to present the Stop the LYE children hair presentation at the 2nd International Hairitage Awards, she was the first to come to mind.

Keianna is truly passionate about – not only caring for the kinks and coils of young ones – but also encouraging them to embrace the beauty in all their natural attributes. She thereby reinforces self-love and self-acceptance. A noble and necessary undertaking.

While diligently managing a busy salon, she also shares knowledge online through her own blog and by being a contributing writer for other online sources. With the wealth of (mis)information available online, it is important to have a competent stylist who can provide accurate information gleaned from years of experience working with all types of hair textures, styles, products and conditions.

I am so very proud to see this wife, mother of 5, salon owner, blogger and writer complete this labor of love. By following the advice in "Coming of Age", I am confident that every young reader of this book can have healthy hair habits, as well as healthy self-esteem.

Ansylla Ramsey
Holistic Hair Care Specialist
International Educator

Introduction

Hello! My name is Keianna. When I was a teenager, I used to hot curl my hair every single day with Vaseline. My favorite hairstyle to wear was flip-curls. The Vaseline gave my hair a perfect shine, and if the wind was blowing outside, my flawless curls didn't move. I was extremely proud for finally mastering a style that made me look beautiful and that was long-lasting. So I thought.

I didn't know until much later that I was known throughout the school as the girl who smelled like burnt hot curlers. I was horrified to have heard this information about myself. I made such an effort to ensure that my hair was trendy, but my attempt was in vain.

I also didn't know until I began to visit a professional hairstylist that my hair was so damaged from scorching it daily that I needed to cut all my hair off completely and start over from scratch. Cutting my hair was a painful, yet necessary, plan to get my hair back on track. After my stylist showed me how to make better choices for my hair, I was able to maintain my hair on my own.

You might be wondering, what led me down the road of frying my hair every day in the first place? No one taught me how to care for my hair properly. My mom perfectly styled my hair until I was in middle school. It felt like once I turned 13, that meant I was old enough to take care of everything concerning my hair all by myself. Not to mention the negative disposition (short, ugly, and nappy) I believed about my hair. The negative thoughts I had concerning my hair led me to a place of, unknowingly, damaging it.

I have a strong feeling that our personal hair stories may have some similarities and being left to our own devices to provide healthy hair and style to our hair with very little information or "know how". I decided to write my book Coming of Age, The Easy Guide to Healthy Hair Care for Teens, because I wanted to provide resources and hair care tips you can do on your own.

This book is a gift from me to you. You no longer have to be stressed out trying to figure out your hair on your own. I believe if you are taught about hair care, you will gain confidence. You will have the information needed to make healthy hair choices that will have long-lasting effects throughout adulthood. By reading my book, you will learn to be better at caring for your hair on your own.

CH 1

Natural Hair Care *for* Teens

You are now a teenager. Many things about you have changed. Your thought process, your body, and feelings about life have matured. You no longer need your parent's/guardian's assistance to care for many of your basic needs; like cleaning up your bedroom, picking out your clothes for school, or choosing your friends. You are mature enough to care for those things yourself.

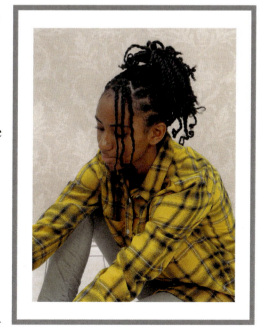

There are many adventures when learning to decide what you like vs. what you dislike. Some experiences from your choices are positive, some negative, but you learn something new from all experiences, which make you a stronger and better person.

Taking care of your hair is the same concept as caring for everything else. Caring for your hair comes with time, practice, making positive choices and seeing results from your hard work. The more you do something correctly; the more your confidence will grow. As your confidence grows, so will your ability to trust your decision-making.

But the questions are, are you currently confident in yourself to care for your natural hair on your own? Why should you properly care for your hair before, during and after wearing protective hairstyles? These are just a couple questions you might be asking yourself. If you can be honest with all of your uncertainties about hair care, you are probably already styling your hair yourself, having more bad hair days than you have good hair days. All that is about to change because this book will give you the inside scoop on caring for your natural hair yourself without having to surf the web, only to be confused by natural hair information written by the novice. This book will give you the advantage to make responsible hair care decisions for yourself.

Before we go any further about healthy hair care, we first have to explore what Natural Hair means? Natural Hair is hair that is unaltered, unprocessed, uncurled, or heat altered hair.

HAIR SCIENCE

Have you ever heard the saying, "people perish due to lack of knowledge"? Let me break down what this saying means in connection with this book. Correct hair care cannot begin without first having an understanding of the hair growing process. This book is in your hand because you want to know how to care for your hair on your own. Don't worry, the inner working of hair growth is broken down in the diagram below.

Hair growth begins from the inside of the body. To get an accurate understanding of the terminologies of hair, we will start from the bottom of the chart and work our way up.

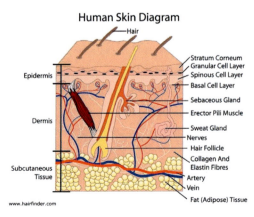

1. Dermal Papilla- Responsible for stimulating hair growth and delivering a constant supply of blood and nourishment to the root.

2. Hair Bulb- The lower expanded extremity of hair. It fits like a cap over the hair papilla at the bottom of the hair follicle. The Hair Bulb is also where hair growth begins.

3. Root- A capping lid over the Dermal Papilla. The hair roots is part of the hair embedded in the hair follicle.

4. Hair Follicle- A small cavity in the epidermis and corium of the skin, from which hair develops.

5. Sebaceous Gland- A small gland that secretes oily matter (Sebum) for lubricating hair and skin.

6. Arrector Pili Muscle- A fan-shaped, smooth muscle which is associated with the base of each hair that contracts. Piloerection, also known as, Goose Bumps.

7. Dermis- A dense inner layer of skin beneath the epidermis. In the area of the Dermis, there are connective tissue, blood vessels, sweat glands, hair follicles, and an elaborate sensory nerve network.

8. Epidermis- The outer, nonvascular and non-sensitive layer of skin, covering the actual skin or corium.

9. Skin Surface- The outer covering of the body.

10. Hair- Slender, thread-like outgrowth of the Epidermis.

11. The Cortex- The middle layer of hair. Inside the hair, there are protein chains that are made up of soft protein which gives hair elasticity and the ability to bend. The Cortex also contains Melanin. It is also the place where chemical change takes place: hair relaxer and or hair color.

12. The Cuticle- The outer protector of the hair with overlapping scales like a fish. The Cuticle is responsible for giving hair shine. It is colorless and thin.

SCALP HEALTH

The Scalp is the barrier between hair growth happening below the skin surface and extending above the skin. The Scalp, is an essential element in the hair care process yet is also one that is most neglected. As a Natural Hair Professional, I've seen horror stories of teenagers not shampooing their scalp/hair for up to 2 to 3 months at a time, trying desperately to save their hairstyle for as long as possible. They are not realizing the scalp is in immediate danger of fungal infections such as ringworm, and yeast-like fungus, just to name a few.

The Scalp has to be cleaned with the same level of importance as cleaning the body. A bad odor comes from the body when the skin isn't washed with soap. The same thing happens when the scalp isn't washed with a cleansing shampoo. If a stinky smell is coming from the direction of your head, it is time to wash your hair with shampoo. Whether your hair is in a natural hairstyle, protective style, boxed braids, crochet braids, or weave style, it is time to take down your hair and shampoo your scalp/hair. If you smell salty sweat coming from your hair, so can everyone else around you. Water and a cleansing shampoo is the only way to deodorize your hair.

HAIR TYPES

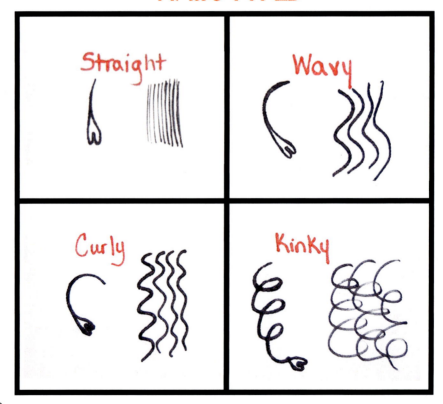

HAIR TEXTURE

Identifying your hair texture is the beginning of hair care. Knowing your hair texture is the guide you'll need that will assist you in providing your hair with the nutrients it needs to thrive and grow. After learning your hair texture, you will be informed of the kinds of techniques and products your hair needs.

1. Straight Hair
2. Wavy Hair
3. Curly Hair
4. Kinky Hair

Most people who "Go Natural" often return with the hopes of having curly hair. It doesn't work like that. Whatever your hair looks like when it is wet is your actual hair texture. What is interesting about hair texture is it is possible to have two to three different hair textures on one head.

When gathering information online about hair texture, you can't trust everything you read. The hair typing chart has grown from four primary type system to a more confusing one. Many of these "systems" have added previously curled hair and hair extension curl patterns to its graph which are not realistic to the hair on a human head while wet. Many natural hair wearers follow The Texture Typing(sm) System and/or The LOIS Hair Typing System. I encourage you to read up on both and decide which hair typing system works best for you. Personally speaking, I follow the traditional Hair Typing System. Hair is either Straight, Wavy, Curly, or Kinky. However, choose whichever system works best for you. That is the beauty of growing up, becoming your own expert and thinking independently.

DIET & HAIR HEALTH

One of the biggest blessings about this stage in your life is the ability to make choices for yourself. These options go far beyond knowing your favorite color and or choosing your friends. You are now beginning to make decisions concerning your lifestyle. Lifestyle choices are often motivated based on how you grew up and your life experiences. Food and eating habits may not seem to be a significant part of a teenager's life, but it is meaningful. What you eat becomes visible on your skin, your body, and how you view yourself. No matter what your lifestyle choices are, **YOU ARE SMART, UNIQUE, and BEAUTIFUL, GIRL!**

We've already discovered thus far that hair care begins from the inside of the body. Before choosing what products are best for your hair, you must first consider your diet and healthy hair lifestyle.

> 1. Omnivore: An individual who eats animal and plant foods.
>
> 2. Clean Eaters: An individual who consumes unaltered and not genetically modified food.
>
> 3. Vegetarian: A person who does not eat meat, fish, fowl, or food derived from animals such as eggs, cheese but subsists on vegetables, fruits, nuts, and grain.
>
> 4. Vegan: A Vegetarian who omits all animal products from the diet.

Hair Care is a total body experience, including drinking water and exercise. Teenagers are recommended according to KidsHealth.org, to have at least an hour of physical activity a day. Whether you join organized sports at school or you walk to school every day, every bit of exercise counts, along with drinking 74.4 oz. of water a day, which equals 8 cups of water.

The eating list above isn't an indicator of one lifestyle choice being better than the other. The list will later assist you in choosing the kinds of hair products that will work for you according to your way of life. Teenagers who live a vegetarian or vegan lifestyle are more than likely going to choose hair products that are holistic and plant-based, while Omnivores and Clean Eaters have the option of using either holistic or mainstream hair products found in the local beauty supply store.

READING PRODUCT LABELS

Before we dive into this discussion on Natural Hair Products, you are probably wondering why learning about hair products is important? It is always important to know what you are placing on your skin. I want to share this one simple fact with you. It isn't a crime to use store bought products on your natural hair. The truth is not everyone can use 100% natural products due to allergies. However, the reason why Natural Hair Stylists, your parents, and natural hair wearers, in general, shy away from using store bought products is that many products on the market have toxic chemicals in them. These toxic chemicals have been proven to make people sick with fibroid disease, cancer, and in some cases caused respiratory diseases. The compounds are added to many of these hair products to preserve shelf life, or are cheap fillers added to the product; with no benefit to hair health and are sold to consumers for the sole purpose of making money. Not every company makes products that are in the best interest of their customer.

If you are curious about what's really in your hair products, visit EWG's Skin Deep Cosmetic Database at www.ewg.org. Turn your hair products over and type in each word in the section of ingredients so you can read for yourself what each word means and how that component will play a factor in your total body health. When you become more aware of what's in your products, you also become aware of what is placed on your skin will be absorbed into your body. Now that I've gotten that out of the way; let's began to explore the mysteries of hair products.

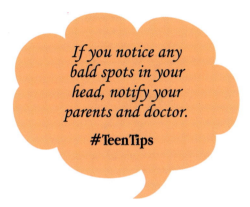

If you notice any bald spots in your head, notify your parents and doctor.

#TeenTips

HAIR PRODUCTS

Here is the topic you all have been waiting for, right? A question people of all ages want answers to, "What Natural Hair Products should I use on my hair?" The answer to this depends on your hair type and your lifestyle. But first, let's talk about the purpose of hair products in general. Hair products sole purpose is to enhance the curl pattern you already have. Knowing your hair texture is the beginning of proper hair care. Knowing this information will guide you in the right direction when you are making hair product purchases that are designed for your hair.

Hair needs both shampoo and conditioner to thrive. The shampoo is used to clean the scalp and hair by opening up the cuticles releasing dirt and buildup from hair. The conditioner is used to soften and restore all nutrients lost during the wash; sealing cuticles back up and locking nutrients inside the hair. Utilizing both shampoo and conditioner helps strengthen the hair shaft, prevents breakage, split ends and hair loss.

Have you ever wondered about the purpose of the hair products needed for everyday beauty? The next list explains the use of each product and its function.

1. Water- Moisturizer, scientifically proven to hydrate the body.

2. Butters- Seals in moisture while preventing brittle hair.

3. Creams- A Light hair lotion that seals in moisture.

4. Pomade- Seals in moisture providing long lasting shine.

5. Mousse- Provides hair with volume, hold and reduces frizz.

6. Oil-Sealant- Not a moisturizer. Locks moisture inside hair

7. Curl Defining Cream- Long-lasting hold and natural curl enhancement.

8. Gel- Holds hair in place

9. Detangler- Untangles hair pain-free.

HAIR GROWTH

Contrary to what is often said, there isn't a hair product that will make your hair grow. Hair products, on the other hand, can assist (along with technique) with maintaining moisture and nutrients into your hair. There isn't a moment where the process of hair care can be neglected, and then grab a bottle of your favorite "miracle grow" and hair growth instantly happens. Wouldn't it be amazing if that could happen? Now here is the truth, hair growth occurs anywhere between six months and six years. Some people's hair grows an inch per month while others have either faster or slower results. Be patient. Everyone's hair growth process is different. Enjoy the journey you are on.

Protein Treatments are designed to recondition and strengthen the hair especially after wearing protective styles which often leaves the hair weak, dry and brittle. Hair care professionals recommend the use of protein treatments every 6 to 8 weeks. There are plenty of Protein Treatment conditioners on the market ranging between $6 -$30 a bottle. Some are in the shape of a soap bar. There are plenty of people who opt out of using store brought Protein Treatments to use eggs and/or mayonnaise to rejuvenate their hair. Healthy hair is strong hair.

> *Not everyone can use holistic products due to allergies. I have a client who has terrible seasonal allergies and cannot use products containing Lemongrass. Teens who are allergic to peanuts should not Shea Butter because Shea Butter is in the nut family.*
>
> **#TeenTips**

PRODUCT SHELF LIFE

The shelf life of hair products is based on their ingredient contents. Products made with raw ingredients have a shorter shelf life, while store bought products that contain non-natural chemicals have a much longer shelf life. Product packaging also plays a role in its lifespan. If there were a war between Jars vs. Pumps, Pumps would win hands down. Jars are more open to contain bacteria/germs due to our hands scooping out product. Germs can also breed from people scooping product with dirty hands and hair left in jars. Always wash your hands before placing them into product jars. Pumps have a protective barrier-the container never opens. Because pump packaging is never opened, there is no way cross contamination would ever exist. Spray bottles and oil containers have the same lifelong fate as Pump packaging.

EXPIRATION DATES

Everything that exists in life has an expiration date. However, there is one fact that must be mentioned, The Federal Drug Administration (FDA) doesn't require hair product makers to have expiration dates or labeling on packaging. Unopened store-bought products (depending on packaging) can last up to 3 years. Once the product has been opened and exposed to the elements, the expiration date decreases by 1 1/2 years. If the product is water-based, the shelf life declines dramatically due to water exposure. For this very reason, it is imperative to purchase products that are packaged in a way with the least amount of exposure to contamination.

The sense of smell is your most prominent defense against spoiled hair products. Having a bad odor isn't a good sign. If the product smells bad, throw it away. If spoiled products are placed on the skin/scalp, a bacterial infection can form. Pimples and rashes on the skin are not cute. Whatever is put on the skin is absorbed into the body. If discoloration and a bad odor are coming from your hair products, it is time to throw them away.

CREATING A REGIMEN

Having a hair care routine creates a regular schedule to ensure your hair gets consistent conditioning, moisture, shine, and cute styles. To ensure success during your hair care regimen, you will need the following: Shampoo, Conditioner, Detangler, and Styling Products.

Hair Care Routines Schedules:
   1. Daily Hair Regimen: Things you do daily to keep your hair healthy.

   2. Weekly Hair Regimen: Apply water and your favorite hair products every couple of days to keep your hair moisturized.

   3. Bi-weekly Hair Regimen: Shampoo, Conditioner, Detangler, Styling Products and New Hair Style.

   4. Monthly Hair Regimen: Shampoo, Conditioner, Detangler, Styling Products and Style. (Hair Extension Methods)

   5. Every Six Weeks Hair Regimen and Protein Treatment.

HOW TO PROPERLY SHAMPOO HAIR

There is a huge difference between shampooing your hair and appropriately shampooing hair. Some girls shampoo their hair but still have dust and dandruff residue on their scalp after washing their hair. Below are steps to follow to help you get the best results from your shampooing experience.

   1. Detangle hair before you use shampoo. This will help you get the best from your shampooing experience.

   2. Adjust the water temperature to warm which opens the hair cuticles.

   3. Allow the water (with the aid of your hands) to rinse all product from scalp

and hair.

4. Apply moisturizing shampoo.

5. Work in the shampoo.

6. Massage the entire scalp first and gently work your way down to the ends of your hair.

7. Repeat

8. Apply your favorite hair conditioner to hair. Let stay for five mins.

9. Rinse Conditioner out with cool water; which closes the cuticles locking moisture from conditioner inside the hair.

> *Be careful when shampooing hair in the shower. Shampoo in the tub can be very dangerous. You can slip, fall, and seriously hurt yourself. If you enjoy washing your hair in the shower, stand on a shower mat in the tub to prevent falls.*
>
> **#TeenTips**

CO-WASHING

Co-washing isn't 100% wrong if done in between washes with shampoo. The purpose of using a moisturizing conditioner is to restore the hair shaft with nutrients lost during the washing. The conditioner is not designed to lift build-up, dirt or debris from hair. Co-washing is not only coating the hair but over time will clog pores on scalp and weigh hair down. Also, if the hair is not properly cleaned with shampoo, the hair will become damaged and break due to suffocation. The purpose of hair care is just that, properly caring for your hair. Cutting corners to seek soft, manageable hair will cause more harm than good in the long run.

LOW MANIPULATION AND PROTECTIVE STYLES: WHAT'S THE DIFFERENCE?

The one main similarity between Low Manipulation and Protective Hair Styling options is the purpose, to protect the hair from breakage. Let's first discuss Low Manipulation Hairstyles. These styles require minimum time to get done. These styles can be changed daily or weekly. Low Manipulation styles are quick styles such as Afro, Afro Puff, Wash N Go, Ponytail, Braid-out, Twist-out, High Buns and Side-Ponytail. Low Manipulation styles do not require the ends to be protected or tucked away.

Protective Hairstyles have a slightly different purpose which is to safeguard the ends of the hair from breakage. The techniques needed to execute protective hairstyles are a little complex and will require more time to do. The following styles are considered Protective Styles: Cornrows, Flat Twists, Double Strand Twists, Braid Updos, Extensions, Crochet Braids, and Wigs. These methods keep the ends of the hair tucked away between two weeks up to six weeks. Hair isn't styled daily.

NIGHT TIME HAIR CARE: DOS & DON'TS

Night time care is paramount because it determines whether you have a good or bad hair day the next morning.

DO'S

1. Do massage temples with castor oil once a week at night.

2. Lightly apply oil to the scalp.

3. Lightly mist hair with water and apply your favorite butter or cream to hair to seal in moisture.

4. Tie hair down with scarf but not super tight. Wearing a tight scarf around your head can contribute to tension and weak edges.

DON'TS

1. Do not put butter, mineral oil or pomade on your scalp. It will clog your pores.

Straight Hair Textures: Avoid Heavy Oil because it will weigh your hair down.
Thick Hair Textures: Your hair is super strong, avoid volumizers.
Kinky Hair Textures: Avoid products with alcohol and heavy gels because it will dry out your hair.

Wavy Hair Textures: Avoid pomades, crunchy or sticky hair gels, and heavy creams.
Curly Hair Textures: Avoid Hair Spray that causes frizz.

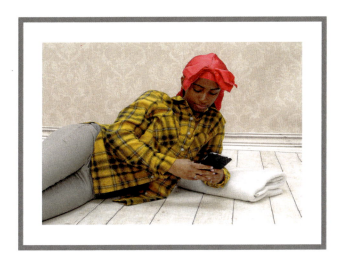

CH 2

Loc Care
for Teens

Locs, a hairstyle dated all the way back to ancient times, are the most beautiful uniquely created hairstyles of Black Culture. Locs are different from most natural hairstyles because wearing Locs is a choice. In the past, Locs weren't widely popular like they are today. Teenagers who choose to wear Locs have a personal expression associated with them. If there is one word to describe Locs, that word would be freedom. To choose a hairstyle that goes against society confinement of what beauty/fashion means is so refreshing. Loc Stars, continue to stand out!

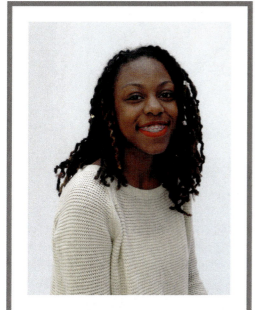

Those who do not understand this cultural hairstyle would ask the question, "What are Locs?" Locs are hair strands that are permanently matted together. Locs are started many different ways, but all have the same result. Freeform Locs are created by allowing the hair to tangle together of its will. Then there are Locs set up in a more organized way such as Palm Rolled which is made by using the palms of the hands. Then there is Latch Hook Locs created using a latch tool with a hook on the ends. Some Locs built from the foundation of gel twist, double strand twist, plaits. The hair parting method of Locs play a huge role in how the Locs mature over time. Although Locs have to be regularly maintained, they grow to long lengths quickly due to low manipulation. These organized tangles have evolved over the years creating an evolution of its own.

LOC CARE, REGIMEN & MAINTENENCE

Most teens who wear Locs have their hair maintained by the hands of a professional or someone they trust. As complex as Locs are, it is understandable if a teenager cannot perform their Loc maintenance themselves. However, it isn't impossible for a teenager to have a regimen they can do on their own. The hair regimen breakdown that's mentioned in chapter one can also be used to build a hair regimen for Locs. Depending on how your Locs were started also determines their care. There is a myth that says in order for your hair to Loc; you are not allowed to wash your hair which is not true. Good hair hygiene practices should always be performed no matter if your hair is in Locs or not. I encourage you to have a hair calendar to keep track of your hair care regimen.

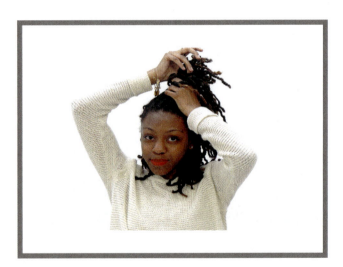

The lessons I share in this book about Locs are recommendations from my experience as a Loctician. As it relates to the kinds of products used to cultivate Locs, less is better. I am going to share with you the same advice I share with my clients. Locs should be shampooed every two weeks or as recommended by your Loctician. Not shampooing your Locs will expose your scalp/hair to nasty disorders and smelly odors. It is recommended to use natural shampoos on Locs to prevent product build-up. Most store bought products approved for Locs are full of mineral oils, petroleum jelly and fillers not good for the hair. Bobeam Natural Hair Products sell 100% natural hair shampoos, specialty oils and hair teas made specifically for Locs, such as the Lemon Drop Shampoo Bar and the Loc Bar. I love these shampoo bars because they clarify the hair and smell amazing. After shampooing and rinsing your hair with water, be sure to get all the shampoo out of your Locs. Follow up with a herbal hair tea blend, and your favorite essential oil blend. All-natural hair products designed for Locs can be purchased at www.bobeamnaturalproducts.com.

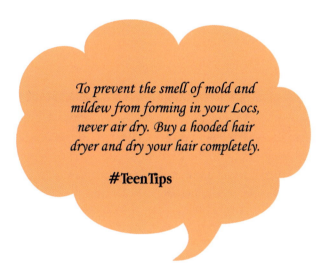

To prevent the smell of mold and mildew from forming in your Locs, never air dry. Buy a hooded hair dryer and dry your hair completely.

#TeenTips

Although someone helps maintain your Locs, you can still moisturize and provide shine to your Locs yourself. Aloe Vera Gel is perfect for Locs. It is light on the hair and is 90% water. We learned in chapter 1 that water is scientifically proven to hydrate the body. Rosewater is awesome for moisturizing and will give your Locs an amazing scent. Rosewater can be purchased at Amazon and your local whole food store. If your scalp needs a natural detox, apple cider vinegar works for some, but my favorite anti fungus treatment is Tea Tree oil. Rice Bran Oil is perfect for Locs. Rice Bran Oil will not leave buildup, is a natural antioxidant, good for sensitive skin, and high in fatty acid. When it comes to the products you put on your Locs, less is always best.

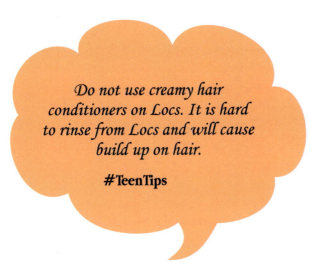

Do not use creamy hair conditioners on Locs. It is hard to rinse from Locs and will cause build up on hair.

#TeenTips

One of the unique qualities about wearing Locs is the 2-in-1 hairstyle options. A Double Strand Twist style can quickly turn into lovely crinkles a few weeks later. To create a fashionable Bobby Pin-less updo style, just put an elastic headband around your head and tuck your Locs into the headband. Locs can be worn in a high bun for a few weeks and turn into yet another super cute crinkle style. Lastly, using Flexi Rods on your Locs will create breathtaking curls. However, be advised, using curling creams or hot curlers should never be used to curl Locs.

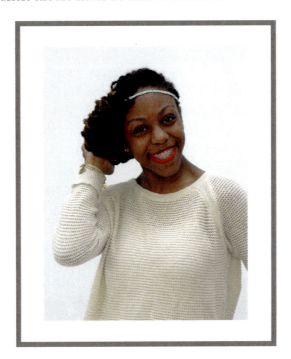

TThe only heat source that can be used to help maintain your Locs is a hooded hair dryer which will be your very best friend while you travel on your Loc journey. If you run out of creative ways to wear your Locs, Loc styles can be worn in the same manner as many Boxed Braid Styles.

Night time care is very simple. Purchase a satin pillow case and wear a Loc scarf to bed. A company that creates beautiful hair garments for Locs is called The Original Loc Soc. To purchase your Loc Soc visit www.soclocsoc.com.

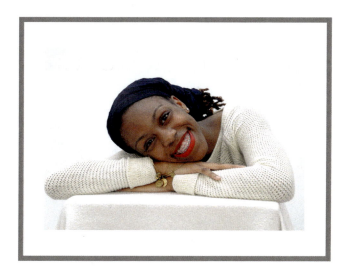

CH 3

Hair Damage: Every Teen's *Nightmare*

He opens the door to your bedroom with only one plan in mind. Tiptoeing, one foot in front of the other. Looking over at you, he sees you sleeping ever so peacefully in bed. You toss from one side of your bed to the next, trying to find your next comfortable position. Suddenly, he drops to the floor and rolls under your bed. EYES POP OPEN! "What was that?" you say to yourself. Five minutes goes by, no sound at all. Heavy eyelids, you fall back to sleep. Easing up

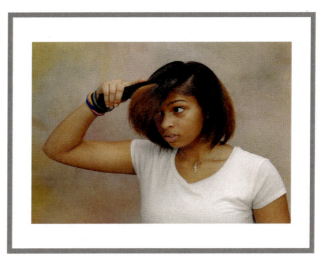

from off the floor, he stands over you lying in bed. Realizing he's got you just where he wants you. With an evil grin, exposing his yellow and brown teeth. Completely unaware of his plan to destroy you. Ending the existence of your edges. Choke the moisture from your hair. He has been damaging your hair for the past forty-five days. The *Bonnet Snatcher* yanks your bonnet off your head and runs out of your room. Popping up out of bed, you touch your head realizing your hair scarf is nowhere in sight.

> *Brushing your hair with 100 strokes makes your hair grow longer is a myth.*
>
> **#TeenTips**

All right, I know that story was a little dramatic, but that is how fast your hair can be damaged. Hair is extremely fragile. Damage can happen literally in a blink of an eye. Below are a few elements that can contribute to hair damage.

- Not Washing Hair
- Heat Damage
- Hair Braiding
- Clip In Extensions
- High Ponytails
- Relaxers
- Over Process Hair Color
- Weave Glue

> *Dropping Flat Irons & Curlers can alter how the equipment works. Never use broken hair styling equipment on your hair. Replace broken tools right away.*
>
> **#TeenTips**

HEAT DAMAGE

It isn't unusual to want to wear your hair straight. You've spent most of your childhood wearing your hair in low manipulation and protective hairstyles. There is nothing wrong with wanting to change up your hair. When it comes to heat styling, it is a catch-22. Whenever heat is added to hair whether it is through hair dryers, flat irons, curlers, silk-presses, or hot comb, your natural curl pattern will be altered. There isn't a way around it. Heat styling straightens your hair. It's important for me to share this information with you so you can count the cost. If you have already made a choice to straighten your hair, it is OK. It isn't a crime to wear your hair straight. Always use a heat protectant. Try to find different ways to preserve your hairstyle, so you don't have to curl your hair every single day.

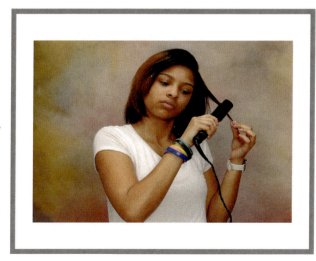

HOW TO PREVENT HEAT DAMAGE

Carrier Oil usage (Castor Oil, Avocado Oil, Coconut Oil, Rice Bran Oil, Olive Oil, Jojoba Oil, Grapeseed Oil and Sweet Almond Oil) is encouraged for different reasons but mainly for its skin and hair nourishing properties. When it comes to heat styling, using carrier oils will scorch your hair. Here is where store-bought product usage is encouraged. Purchasing heat protecting serums, creams, and sprays will save your hair from being burned from flat ironing and hot curling. Using a heat protectant should always be used during heat styling.

SAFE HEAT STYLING TEMPERATURES

This Heat Styling Chart was inspired by Thirstyroots.com

Hair Type:	Thin to Fine	Normal to Medium	Coarse
Hair Temperature:	Below 360(F)	360-390(F)	360-410(F)

"Healthy hair begins to melt and burn at 451 degrees (F)." Thirstyroots.com

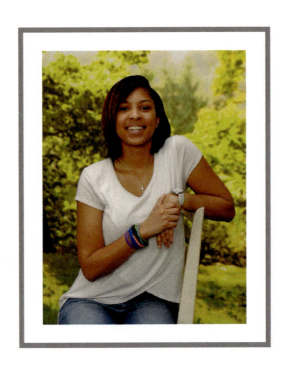

CH 4

Trendy Braids
&*Their Care*

Wearing hair in cornrows, braids, weaves, and clip-in hair extensions has been a staple in Black History and Culture for centuries. Many of the styles you see people wearing in their hair today are timeless and created by our African Ancestors. There is nothing new under the sun as it relates to hair braiding. Trends come and go with time and return.

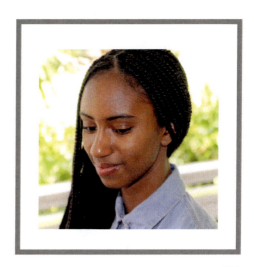

WHY BLACK GIRLS LOVE HAIR EXTENSIONS

Teenage girls love wearing their hair in extensions. Hair extensions provide styling versatility, experimentation with many styling options, lengths, and colors which also allow each person to fashion their hair according to their unique personality. Hair Extensions are perfect for any occasion. They can be pinned up, worn straight, curly, kinky and wavy. When inspired, teenagers sometimes mimic hairstyles of their favorite celebrities. Let's face it; hair extensions are a ton of fun. These hairstyles allow teens to look and feel beautiful without daily manipulating their natural hair.

BEING YOURSELF WHILE WEARING EXTENSIONS

One of the first things people see after looking into your face is your hair. It's no wonder every young woman wants their hair to be fashionably perfect to match their beautiful face. I know when I was your age, when my hair was freshly done, I felt confident. I didn't mind having all eyes on me when I walked into a room. Wearing hair extensions is slightly different from wearing your real hair and can sometimes take on a life of its own. Some teens feel more comfortable and confident wearing hair extensions than wearing their natural hair especially if their natural hair is shorter than their peers. Girls your age often look older when wearing hair extensions which can sometimes make them act older than they are. It is critical that you be yourself no matter what hairstyle you choose to wear. You are fabulous with or without hair extensions.

> *One of many contributions to an itchy scalp while wearing hair extensions is a chemical compound called Alkaline. Alkaline is added to Kanekalon-synthetic hair to preserve it while it sits on store shelves for weeks, months and years preventing hair from molding. It's also flame resistant.*
>
> **#TeenTips**

BRAIDING CARE

Now that you are older and are contemplating wearing your hair in a "protective hairstyle" using hair extensions. It is important not to think of the result of solely having a cute hairstyle. Transitioning your thoughts from fashionable hair to overall hair care can be a lot of information to process at one time. You were unaware of the importance of scalp/hair maintenance when wearing protective styles. You never really had to think about maintaining your hair until now. But all that is about to change. The information provided in this book was written with you in mind. You will be knowledgeable by the end of this book of what it takes to maintain your hair on your own.

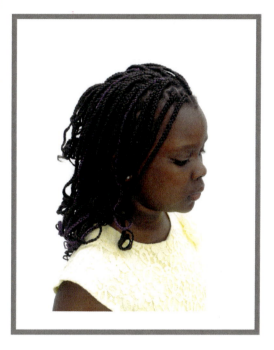

IS THAT ODOR COMING FROM YOUR HEAD?

Last year, I hosted a Teen Hair Chat Focus Group Event at my home. During the conversation, I asked the girls a question, "Have you ever encountered a situation where you smelled a bad odor coming from your braids, weave, or crochet braids?" Four out of the six teens answered yes. I wasn't shocked by their answer because I was once a teenage volleyball player. Let's just say, my braids did not smell like fresh lavender after practice.

Here are four reasons why hair extensions have a bad odor.
1. Teens forget to shampoo scalp/hair before receiving a hair extension installation.

2. Teens are leaving extensions in hair longer than four to six weeks.

3. Sweat is forming and then drying over the course of days, weeks, and months from physical activities.

4. Applying excessive amounts of product to scalp/hair contributing to buildup.

IS YOUR SCALP SAYING, "SHAMPOO ME PLEASE?"

Deodorizing your hair by shampooing before, during and after a hair extension installation is imperative. A clean scalp isn't itchy or sweaty. Clean hair is free of debris and not to mention how great your scalp feels and how wonderful your hair smells. Don't be scared to shampoo your hair. Clean hair equals healthy hair.

> *Do not use fingernail glue of any kind to install braids or weaves in your hair. Your real hair will be damaged.*
>
> **#TeenTips**

BRAIDING CARE & REMOVAL

Individual Braids & Twist Estimated Installation Time: between 4 to 8 hours. Estimated Leave-In Time: 4 to 6 weeks.

Braid removal means the elimination of hair extensions either single braids and twists. Here is what you will need to remove extensions from your hair safely.

1. Clip the ends with scissors.

2. Use the rattail comb point to take down the braids from ends to roots carefully.

3. Once the braid is out, examine your natural hair.

4. If there is build up (dirt) near the roots of your hair, loosen up the hair in that area with your fingertips and break up the buildup.

5. Take the spray bottle & mist your hair with water.

6. Take an Afro Comb and comb the area where the buildup was.

7. Remove shed hair and buildup.

8. Continue to follow these steps until hairstyle is completely taken down.

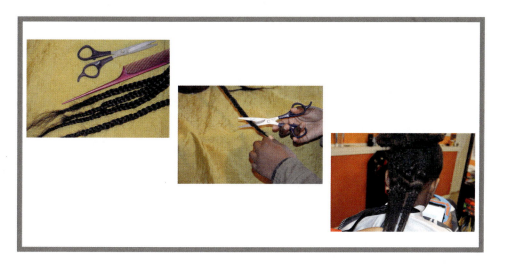

WEAVE REMOVAL
Installation Time: 2-4 hours
Leave-In Time: 4 to 6 Weeks.

A hair weave can be installed into the hair two different ways; glued or sewn which also determines how the hair extensions should be taken down. The way you choose to wear your hair is an essential part of your creative expression. However, I do not like the idea of installing a weave using glue. Using weave glue may appear to be the quickest way to get luxurious flowy hair, but weave glue is a very toxic latex. It can cause allergic reactions to those who are allergic to latex.

No matter how cautious you are with avoiding weave glue contact with your hair; there is always a possibility of the adhesive coming in touch with your real hair. This glue can cause damage to your scalp suffocating it by covering it completely and break your hair completely off. I have seen friends and family who had to cut parts of their hair because there were sections of glue stuck to their hair.

It is far better to have your weave sewn in than glued in, but the choice is yours. Choose whichever option is right for you.

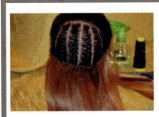
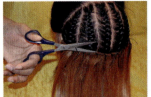
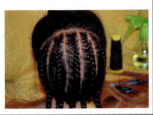

Here is how you can remove a Sew N Weave.

1. Use your fingers to locate the thread.

2. Use a pair of scissors or a seam ripper to cut a piece of thread.

3. Unravel thread.

4. Takedown tracks or weave.

5. Repeat the process until all the weave hair is removed.

6. Then, take a spray bottle filled with water and spray your cornrows.

7. Take the rat-tail comb and take down your cornrows.

8. Detangle your whole head with a wide tooth comb before shampooing.

CROCHET BRAIDS REMOVAL
Installation Time: 1-3 hours
Leave-In Time: 2 to 4 weeks

Removing Crochet Braids from your hair is much different than removing boxed braids and or weave. Crochet braids are installed into your previously braided cornrows using a latch hook tool. One wrong move during the take down process will have you missing a huge chunk of hair. It is crucial to take down your crochet braids carefully. Next are the steps to removing Crochet Braids without cutting your natural hair.

1. Open the hair and locate cornrows.

2. Take scissors and carefully cut the crochet hair close to the knot.

3. Remove crochet hair away from cornrows.

4. Continue the removal process until all hair has been taken out.

5. Then, take a spray bottle filled with water and spray your cornrows.

6. Take the rat-tail comb and take down your cornrows.

7. Detangle your whole head with a wide tooth comb before shampooing.

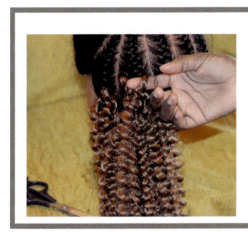
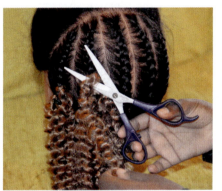

WEARING WIGS

Installation Time: 5 minutes
Leave-In Time: Taken Off Nightly

Wearing a wig is probably the easiest form of hair extensions. It is easier because the hair is taken off nightly. It is easy to maintain your natural hair underneath because you can still continue your hair regimen to ensure your natural hair remains healthy. But wigs also have the potential to damage your hair. Most wigs are sold with a small comb in the front and the back of the wig. Regularly placing the wig comb in the area of your hairline day after day can cause tension and pull your hair out. I recommend wearing a wig for one week or when you are having a bad hair day. I would not recommend wearing a wig for two weeks or more especially if your hairline is damaged.

WEARING EXTENSION: PROS & CONS

PROS:
1. Wearing hair extensions are perfect for protecting your hair from daily manipulation.
2. You have the ability to wake up and go with very little thought about how you will wear your hair.
3. It is easy to shampoo and blow dry with no worries about style.

CONS:
1. Tight hair extensions will pull your hair out.
2. Extensions left in the hair longer than 6 to 8 weeks will damage hair.
3. Dry hair due to lack of shampooing, Conditioning, and Care.
4. Getting Extensions installed back to back without taking a rest will break your hair off.
5. Causes the hairline to bald.
6. Excessive pulling will cause a sore and tender scalp.
7. Weaken natural hair.

Taking care of your real hair before, during and after wearing hair extensions is vital. Neglecting your hair will cause a lifetime of issues. These issues can be prevented if the proper hair care steps are executed from beginning to the end on a consistent basis.

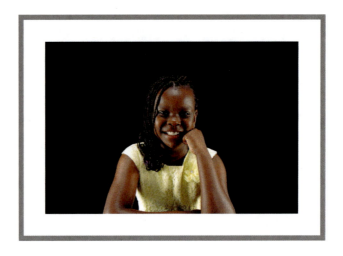

CH 5

Protecting *Your* Edges

What happened to your edges? Are they on vacation? The jokes online are endless ridiculing thin, broken edges. Recently, there was a hashtag circulating entitled #NoEdges, and of course, the memes were hilarious. I've chuckled at a few myself. Not to mention reading stories about our favorite celebrities with broken edges underneath their braids and hair weaves. But having thin edges isn't funny to the many teenagers who suffer from balding. The conversation of

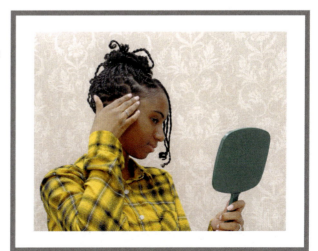

having broken edges is a very uncomfortable subject. Whether spoken or unspoken, hair that recedes backward is noticeable because it is so close to the face. If teenagers who suffer from this condition could find a magic product to help them instantly grow their hair back, they would purchase it in a heartbeat. I see why so many kids are insecure about their edges, especially those teens whose hair will never grow back or was lost due to a medical condition. They will have to accept the fact that things for them will not change, as well as find a way to mask the problem, so they will not be made fun of by their peers.

WHAT ARE EDGES?

Many people call the hair around the face "edges". However, the proper term is a hairline. According to WebMD.com, the hairline is hair that grows around the outline of the head, especially across the front. The hair in the area of the hairline is soft, which is why most people call it "baby hair." The hair in this area isn't as long or as strong as the hair on other parts of the head. We have to be careful with how we handle the hair around our face.

> *Be mindful of how tight your hair bonnet is on your head at night. Any form of tension from your hair scarf can cause the hairline to become weak.*
>
> #TeenTips

PUBLIC ENEMY #1: TENSION

One of the biggest menaces that attack the hairline of Black girls and women is too much tension. People wear tight cornrows, tight braids, tight twists, tight weaves, and uncomfortable wigs on their heads. Tension hairstyles are painful, makes the scalp tender, forms pustules (tiny red or white bumps near hairline) and give you a headache. It seems that no matter how many hair professionals speak on talk shows or are featured in magazines discussing the risk factors of hair tension, the facts are ignored. The worst part is the result is always the same, hair loss. Next are a few causes of why many people edges are broken or completely nonexistent.

1. Not using proper hairstyling tools.

2. Constantly brushing sides with a hard bristle brush.

3. Applying Edge Control to the hair daily.

4. Consistently wearing tight protective hairstyles.

5. Braiding every piece of baby hair into the style (cornrows, braids, etc.)

6. Leaving hairstyles in for extended periods of time collecting dirt and crusted product buildup.

PUBLIC ENEMY #2: EDGE CONTROL

I completely understand why a lot of teenagers are obsessed with perfect edges. Beautifully laid edges make a hairstyle look polished. However, applying too much edge control can break the hair off. Edge control is a sticky gel that hardens the hair to make it lay flat and stay in one place. This product contains alcohol, which has been proven to dry out hair, making the hair brittle. It also makes the hair crunchy. Natural hair thrives when moisturized. Dry and brittle hair will break.

I am not trying to scare you away from using edge control altogether but moderation is the key. For best results, begin your regimen at night. Get a spray bottle and mist your edges with water first. Apply a small amount of edge control to your hairline. Use a soft bristle brush and gently brush your sides down. Tie a scarf around your hair firmly but not too tight. Doing this at night will ensure your hair wil lay down by morning. Also, do not apply edge control to your hair every day. Just mist the area where edge control was used with water, and lightly brush the hair with a soft bristle brush.

> *Many people do not take care of their health until a problem arises, and then they want to go to the doctor. The same scenario happens in hair care. No one takes hair care seriously until a problem occurs and then they visit a hairstylist. To prevent hair loss in the area of the hairline will take daily effort.*
>
> **#TeenTips**

HAIR LOSS PREVENTION: SAVING OUR EDGES

Hair loss prevention is all about eliminating risk factors before the problem begins. If there is a strategy in place to protect the hair around the hairline, the risk factors for balding are reduced. Here are a few key points that will assist you in creating a strategy to fight against hairline hair loss.

1. Follow your weekly or bi-weekly hair care regimen.

2. Moisturize hair with water, cream, and seal in the moisture with oil.

3. Add variety to your style with low manipulation and protective hair styling.

4. Do not cornrow, braid, or twist your edges during the hair styling process.

5. Protect your hairline by sleeping with a satin bonnet or scarf at night.

Following the hair tips listed above will ensure healthy hair and reduce hair loss near your hairline. Healthy hair begins from the inside of your body to the outside. Whatever you put into your body will show up on the outside of your body. Eat right and drink plenty of water. Also, every few days gently massage your edges with

Castor Oil. Castor Oil is rich in fatty acids such as Ricinoleic Acid, Oleic Acid, Linoleic Acid, A-Linoleic Acid, Stearic Acid, Palmitic Acid and Dihydroxystearic Acid. Castor Oil is also a Humectant that retains moisture to the skin.

EDGES: GROWTH AFTER DAMAGE

Growth after damage depends on why the hair in the area of your hairline came out. If your hair falling out is genetic, you will have to consult with your doctor and ask what are the best ways to grow your hair back in the area of your hairline. If your hair is thinning due to excessive hair stying, you would have to give your hair a break from adding any additional hair to your head, meaning, no braids, weaves, wigs at least for three months. Began by finding low manipulation styles you can do on your own. Please note, if there is no hair in the area of hair loss, there is a chance that your hair will never grow back. But if there is a little bit of fuzz there, there is a chance your hair will grow again. To be sure of the state of your natural hair, consult your doctor and or visit a professional stylist.

CH 6

Styling *Tools* & Accessories

It is impossible to create a new hairstyle without considering styling tools. Styling tools will assist you in executing the style you are trying to accomplish. Below is a list of styling tools you will need to style your hair yourself. All equipment can be purchased at your local beauty supply store (online) for reasonable prices and in a variety of colors. Have fun shopping for your new styling tools.

HAIR TOOLS

1. Afro Pick: Used to comb out Afro Hair.

2. Wide tooth comb: A wide tooth comb assists in detangling wet or dry hair.

3. Evolve First Line Rat-tail Comb: This comb is used to part hair for styling, oiling, and braiding.

4. Pin-tail Comb: The pin-tail comb use is for hair parting. (also called a rat-tail comb)

5. Dual-sided Military Brush: This brush works best on long and short hair. The soft bristle side used on edges and short hair. The hard bristle side is for long hair.

6. Teasing Comb: The teasing comb is used to give flat hair weight and volume; to look bigger.

7. Double Prong Clips: Are multifunctional. This clip is used to secure hair in place, Loc maintenance, hair setting, pin curls, volumizes hair.

8. Bobby Pins: Bobby Pins are commonly used to pin hair in place.

9. Butterfly Clamps: Designed to keep hair away from the face while styling. Wide teeth prevent hair breakage from snagging.

10. Paddle Brush: Designed for straight hair with cushion bristles for scalp massage.

11. Flex Rods: Flex Rods are soft twist rollers designed to give you the perfect curls with minimum to no heat.

12. Perm Rods: Are also multifunctional. They are used to set hair and curl the ends of braid styles.

13. All-Purpose Comb: Is a multipurpose comb that works well with all hair textures.

14. Felicia Leatherwood Brush: Hair Detangling Brush.

15. Volume Brush: Designed to create volume.

16. Spray Bottle: Add water or your favorite hair moisturizers to spray on your hair.

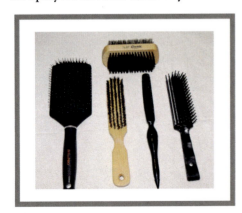
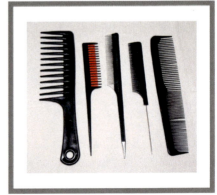

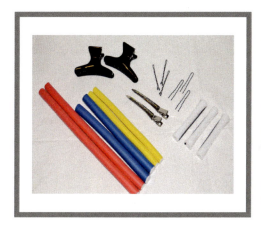
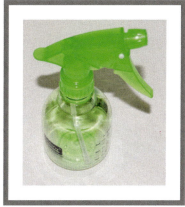

HOW TO CLEAN STYLING TOOLS

Clean styling tools aren't always on the forefront of the mind when rushing to get to school on time. Cross contaminating old, dirty hair left in combs, and brushes, and using them on clean hair has now made your hair a mess. Cleaning hair supplies is a must. If your combs and brushes are for personal use, you can get away with using shampoo to clean your styling tools quickly. However, if you are sharing your styling tools with family members and friends, bacteria can be spread from person to person. Styling tools must be adequately cleaned with an antiseptic to prevent the spread of infectious disease.

Antiseptic means free from or cleansed of germs and other microorganisms. Antiseptics can be safely used on the skin. Accordong to Dictionary.com, Listerine, Alcohol, Witch Hazel and Sea Breeze are all antiseptics. Sanitize your hair tools by first removing all hair and debris, wash them with hot , soapy water, rinse thoroughly and dry. Alcohol wipes are perfect to clean your metal hair clips. You can also use alcohol to clean the outside of your spray/product bottles to cut down on handling greasy products.

HAIR BONNET

The hair bonnet is used for hair health and protection. The hair bonnet keeps hair moisturized and helps the hairstyle last longer. Just like hair is subjected to product build-up and dirt, so is the hair bonnet. Depending on the quality of your hair bonnet, it should either be hand washed, or machine washed once a week in a mesh bag. Wearing a clean bonnet on your head at night is refreshing.

HAIR ACCESSORIES

Hair accessories can make an ordinary hairstyle bold, colorful and unique. Hair accessories are not only for little kids. There are plenty of accessories created specifically for teenagers so don't be afraid to wear them. Below are a few hair accessories I think you will love.

1. Headbands with or without the comb.

2. Hair Combs.

3. Bun Makers.

4. Ponytail Creators.

5. Loc Jewelry.

6. Zodoca Magic Hair Twist.

7. The Puff Cuff Hair Clamp.

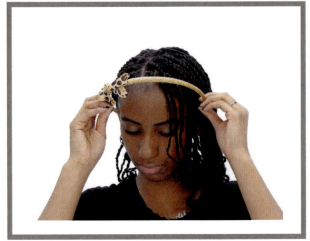

Just like your hair and bonnet should be cleaned regularly, so should hair accessories, especially cloth headbands and bows. To clean your hair accessories without damage, place all hair accessories in a mesh bag. Wash on delicate cycle and allow your hair accessories to air dry. Do not put hair accessories in the dryer. Mesh bag can be purchased at your local craft store.

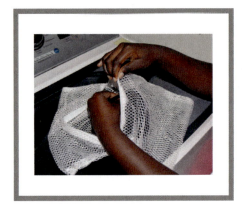
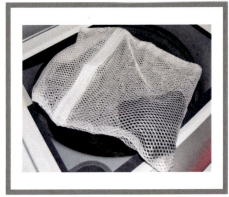

CH 7

Should Friends Style *Your* Hair?

One of the best things to do as a teenager is spending quality time with friends. Friends are loving, understanding and fun to be around. It isn't unusual to bond with friends doing girly things like nails, make-up, having in-depth discussions and styling one anothers hair. "A friend is someone who gives you total freedom to be yourself," Jim Morrison. Your friends understand you and your style inside out.

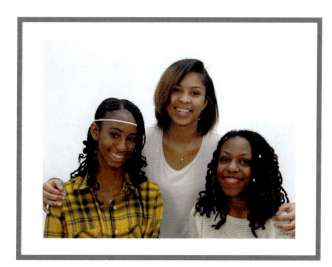

There is a difference between teens who love to style hair and those who will do it because they are asked. Some teenagers can style hair very well but due to lack of knowledge, do not

47

have an understanding of how to provide love and care to the scalp and hair. For instance, what does it mean to be heavy handed? Braiding hair too tight can damage your hair. However, so many teenagers follow the philosophy that is often taught in the Black Community that wearing tighter braids looks better and last longer.

> *There is nothing wrong with allowing your friends to style your hair in less elaborate hairstyles. However, anything that would compromise the hairline, your nap, your scalp, or using unsanitized hair styling tools would not be in the best interest of your hair health.*
>
> **#TeenTips**

Let's also consider other factors. Many teenagers see the process of styling hair and sometimes assume it is easy and in most cases hairstyling is easy. But hairstyling isn't solely about the hair. The scalp, hair follicle, hair shaft and overall health of the hair must also be considered.

Allowing peers to style your hair can be hit or miss depending on their skill level. Many teenagers begin their hair styling career in high school during cosmetology school. Then, there are other times where teens learn proper hair styling techniques from a family member who works in the beauty industry. So, if you are asking yourself this question, "Should my friends style my hair?" consider the skill level of your buddies. Don't forget to keep your eyes on how attractive their hair looks. Ask questions and be very observant. If a person doesn't know how to care for their hair, they won't do a great job caring for your hair.

CH 8

When To Seek *A* Professional

It is great to have a professional stylist in your life, primarily one who specializes in hair care. They are here to educate you on all your hair care needs. I love providing my clients with hair styling options that work best for their hair and showing them how to execute styles at home. Visiting a hair professional regularly or quarterly will ensure your hair stays healthy.

Checking in with your hairstylist will correct any mistake made while at home. Everyone makes mistakes. If you've made any errors in your hair care journey, your professional hairstylist will share accurate information while using correct methodologies in the event any problems may have arisen.

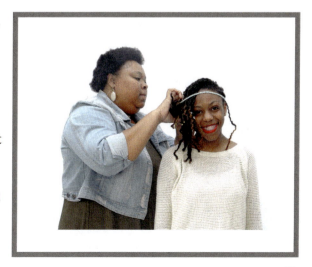

> *If you decide to visit a professional hairstylist, be sure to write down all of your concerns about your hair on a notepad. Submit concerns to your stylist to get the conversation started. Your stylist will give you honest advice and take great care of your hair.*
>
> **#TeenTips**

It is necessary to find a hair care professional for the following reasons to ensure your hair remains healthy:

1. Chemical processes: relaxer, hair color, hair treatments.

2. Thermal Straightening Systems: Blowout, Silk Press.

3. Loc Installation: Sisterlocs(TM), Starter Locs, Loc Repair.

4. Hair Cut: Professional Hair Cuts and Trims.

5. Individual Braids: Braid Install and Braid Removal.

Heat styling can be very tricky. Hair Experts will provide the proper heat protection and temperature during styling. If you are planning to get a silk press or flat iron from a professional, make sure the stylist has a Cosmetology License as well as have references to past client results on their website. There are some dishonest people promoting services they are not qualified to do. Make sure you do your research.

> *Visit a doctor if you have an incredible itch on the scalp, signs of fungus on hair/scalp, had direct contact with chemicals in eyes/skin, burned by hot water during braid install, or burned by hot curlers.*
>
> **#TeenTips**

You will also need a expert stylist for quarterly consultations, top-notch hair extension installation, styles for special occasions and advice on professional products you can use on your hair at home. If you are concerned about high-cost salon visits, with help from your parents, save your money and create a plan when to visit a stylist. Having healthy hair should be a long-term goal and is just as important as taking care of your mind, body, and spirit. Your hair is a significant part of your identity. Weigh your options. If you maintain your natural hair properly at home, you will only need to visit a hair professional seasonally, four times a year, which cuts down the cost dramatically. Allow professional advice to be your guide.

CH 9

Be Encouraged!

I know this was a lot of information to take in. Starting something new all by yourself can be hard. There will be days you will forget to rinse all the shampoo from off your scalp, or days you do not want to start the process of your regimen. There will be days you will experience bad hair days, and there will also be the times you are very successful in accomplishing your hair care goals. Your journey will be filled with peaks and valleys, but every experience is a learning experience. So, don't be hard on yourself. Importantly, don't give up.

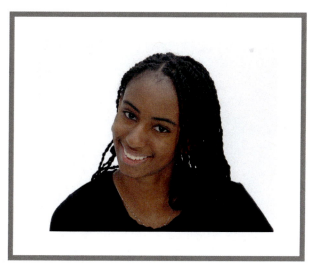

You can do anything you set your mind to do. The good news is you already know what you like and dislike about your hair. Practice until you master your goal...it is all about planning and executing what you want to do. You can do it! And remember, once you learn something, nobody can take that information away from you. I am already proud of you for taking steps towards bettering yourself. Celebrate yourself and be confident. You are so DOPE! Very soon your hair will be the life of the party. You are the perfect advocate for your hair.

Take charge and SOAR!

CH 10

Your Hair Diary

DOCUMENTING YOUR HAIR JOURNEY!

GLASSES OF WATER PER DAY

Sunday	Monday	Tuesday	Wednesday	Thursday	Friday	Saturday

MULTI-VITAMINS

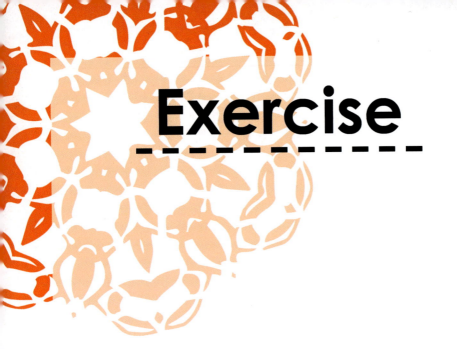

Exercise

Hair Regimen Day

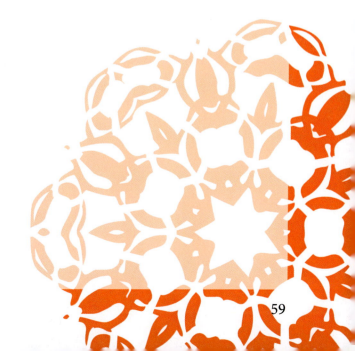

Picture Collage
of your
Favorite Hairstyles

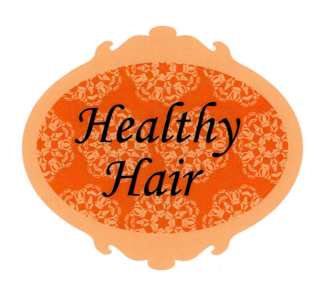

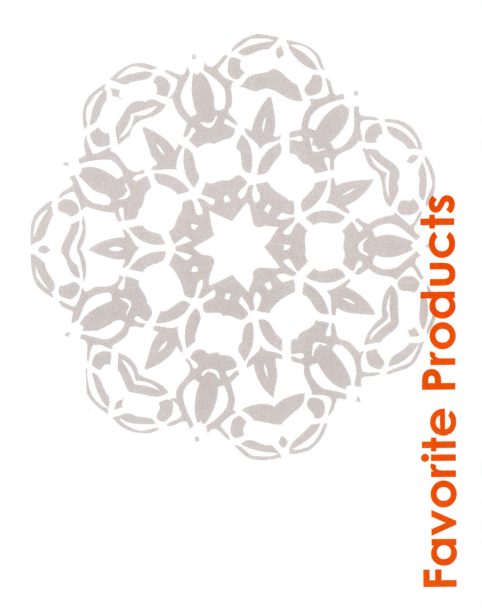

Favorite Products

Must-Have Hair Styling Tools

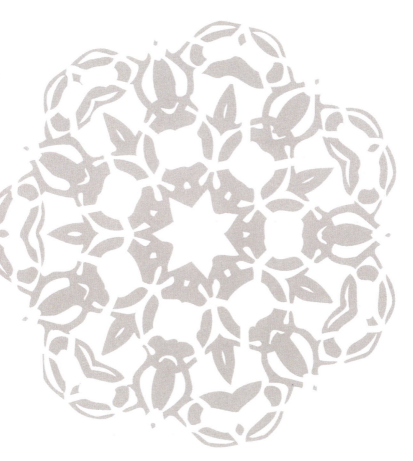

Favorite Protective Styles

Favorite Low Manipulation Styles

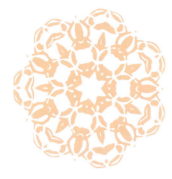
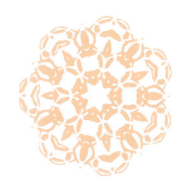
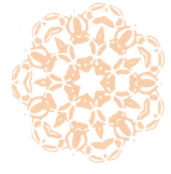
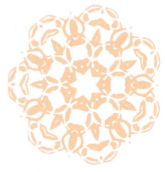

Hair Trimming Schedule

DATE	DESCRIPTION OF HAIR TRIM

Hair Tips
from your Stylist

What Have You *Learned* About Your Hair?

Acknowledgments

God, You have walked with me through every journey my entire life. Thank you for your love, your Word, protection and for answering my prayers. I love you.

To my husband, words cannot express how much you mean to me. Your love towards me is real. I see it in your actions daily. Your support is why I can fulfill my dreams. I love your soul. My heart is yours forever.

To my children, Raequan, Aaron, Adrian, Brooke & Brielle: Thank you for supporting me in hair shows, photo shoots, keeping my studio tidy, being on your best behavior while I work with clients from home. You are my little army. I love you from the bottom of my heart. May all your dreams come true.

To my inner circle: Thank you, mom, for speaking into my life. For motivating me and for being a prayer warrior on my behalf. I am thankful to call you mom. Ms. Myra, I love you. Thank you for supporting my family. Katrina and Stephanie, thank you for being a listening ear and motivator. Love you, Girls. Nick and Kisha, thank you for always being #TeamKeianna. I love you guys. Stacy Cook, from the beginning, you were a believer of my dream. Thanks for being a sister from another mother. I love you, Stacia and Tyra. Bridgett, thanks for traveling to New York and for attending hair industry events with me. Your support means a lot. Angie & Gabby, thanks for the girls' time we share. I love you.

To Stacey Taylor owner of The Sistah Cafe, and Our Natural Kids: Since 2010, you took a chance with an amateur writer and allowed me to join your team. I have grown tremendously as a writer over the years. I thank you from the bottom of my heart for being a genuine person and friend. I love you & Little Chick.

Marcia Kargbo, you are amazing. I will forever remember the day you sat in my chair to get your hair done and how you poured words of wisdom into my life. I salute you.

Special Thanks to the champions who help bring this project to life: Ansylla Ramsey, Olivia Thompson, Julian B. Kiganda, Adeea Rogers, Ms. Deirdre, Aja, Jayln, Jada, Brooke, Brielle, Shelby Tuck-Horton, Laquita Thomas, Amber Muhammad, and the staff at Portrait Innovations Waldorf. Thank you for your time, positive energy and for supporting me with one of the biggest milestones of my life. I couldn't have done this without you.

To Gloria Erickson and the entire London Lane Designs and Publishing staff, this opportunity you have given me to produce this book will never leave my heart. A dream I had with me since I was a little girl was made possible through you. May God continue to bless you. Thanks, from the bottom of my heart.

Last, but not least, To My Chi Chi Sophistication Kids Natural Hair Studio Tribe, We were once strangers and have grown together as a family. You trust me. You took a chance with me when nobody knew my name. You scheduled hair appointments and left my studio with a smile. This book is for you. Big things are happening at Chi Chi Sophistication Kids Natural Hair Studio, and it all began with you. I love you. Thank You for Everything.

Resources

Research
Teen Focal Group: Chi Chi Sophistication Kids Natural Hair Studio Clients. www.chi-chi-sophistication.com

Websites
TheSistahCafe.com
WebMD.com
EWG Skin Deep www.ewg.org
Thirstyroots.com

Books
Milady Standard Natural Hair Care And Braiding by Diane Carol Bailey
The Knotty Truth by M. Michele George.

Photo Credits
Photography Portrait Innovations Waldorf: Associates Sheryl C and Derrick C. Shelby-Tuck-Horton and Keianna Johnson

This book was written independently and was not endorsed by any brand listed in this book.

About *the* Author

Keianna (KeeKee) Johnson is the owner of Chi Chi Sophistication Kids Natural Hair Studio, Specializing in Natural Hair and Braiding for Children ages 2-17, www.chi-chi-sophistication.com. Keianna provides signature braid styles for all occasions.

Certified in Natural Hair and Braiding through Madam Walker's Braidery and Schools. An Award winning hairstylist, Keianna received the prestigious Master's Pioneer Award in 2015 and won The Natural Hair Award, Children's Stylist of The Year, for two consecutive years in a row.

With a passion for writing, Keianna is the Social Information Contributor for Our Natural Kids: Parents online resource center promoting natural hair health, style, and maintenance for Kids. Children Natural Hair Care Advocate, Speaker, and Blog Contributor for The-SistahCafe.com. Keianna also writes weekly on her site KeiannaJohnson.com.

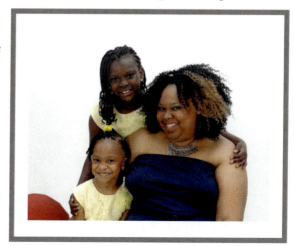